101 BEST PYRAMID TRAINING WORKOUTS

THE ULTIMATE CHALLENGE WORKOUT COLLECTION

STEWART SMITH, CSCS, USN (SEAL)

101 BEST PYRAMID TRAINING WORKOUTS

Text Copyright © 2020 Stewart Smith

Library of Congress Cataloging-in-Publication Data is available.
ISBN: 978-1-57826-858-0

Book design by Carolyn Kasper

10 9 8 7 6 5 4 3 2 1
Printed in the United States

CONTENTS

PREPPING FOR PYRAMID WORKOUTS

T he pyramid.

A warmup, max out and cooldown all rolled into one, the pyramid workout is referred to by many as "the perfect workout". The typical pyramid describes an "active rest" circuit of exercises (resting while doing other exercises) and is a great foundation builder for increasing endurance and muscle stamina. It is also a muscle growth workout—with calisthenics and high volume style resistance training, pyramid workouts are a great way to build mass.

The 100 stand-alone workouts in this book are among my favorite pyramid workouts I have ever created. These are my top 100 individual workouts that focus mainly on calisthenics, running, swimming, rucking, and easy-to-use weights like dumbbells, kettlebells, and sandbags. These are mostly high volume workouts, but you will see some heavy weight reverse pyramids, speed pyramids, and even swimming pyramids of different varieties, all of which are a testament to the versatility and ease with which pyramid workouts can be inserted into virtually any routine.

I recommend these workouts be performed two to three times a week for the upper body, with lower body and cardio pyramids in between as needed or desired. Just make sure to change things up with the many workouts included in this book—adding variety to your workout regimen is a surefire way to avoid plateaus and keep improving.

Rules of the PT Pyramid

1. Don't do it every day. Unless you change up the exercises you're doing—focusing on your upper body one day and your lower body the next—the kind of volume of repetitions involved in pyramid workouts will require you take a day off before working the same muscle group again.

2. Don't go crazy with it. When you fail at an exercise, either change that exercise to an easier version, or else start to work your way back down the pyramid in reverse order. You can build up to some crazy high volume with these workouts and not even realize it, especially on legs and core exercises. Make sure you're progressing smartly: don't do 100 pull-ups in a single workout if you have never done more than 15–25 reps at once.

3. Get creative with it That said, you can—and should—get creative with adding exercises, reps and multiples to let you push yourself without hurting yourself. Adding a diverse group of exercises to your routine is fun and allows the body to recovery with active. For example, you may find that core exercises serve as good rest activity.

HOW TO USE THIS BOOK

The workouts in this book are organized into sections based on the type of workout they offer: upper body, upper body calisthenics and cardio, lower body calisthenics and cardio, full body calisthenics/resistance and cardio, and cardio/mobility workouts. Within these sections, each workout is given a descriptive moniker so that you can easily select the best workout for each day.

Some workouts are quick, while others require at least an hour to complete. Regardless, your goal should be to do what you can on that day and arrange your workouts smartly.

My advice on arranging the workouts into a complete week (5-6 days of training) would be as follows:

- Do your upper body workouts on Monday, Wednesday, and Friday. You can also add in cardio workouts after the upper body resistance workouts. (Cardio is often mixed into these particular workouts.)

- Add leg days on the days in-between your upper body regimens (Tuesday, Thursday, and Saturday) or at least some form of cardio where you use your legs, such as running, biking, rucking, swimming (with fins), or rowing.

- Given this type of volume—even in calisthenics—it is recommended you use the same muscle group *every other day* when it comes to resistance training to allow for maximum recovery and growth. (The other option is to focus on full body workouts and do them every *other* day of the week, with rest or cardio days in between. Cardio pyramids have been provided for those days as well.)

- Progress your cardio workouts logically up to several days per week of running, biking, and swimming, but keep rucking at two to three times per week max for the purposes of these workouts.

The rules are that simple!

NOTE: There are no exercise descriptions or visual breakdowns provided for these workouts. If there are any exercises you do not recognize, see my YouTube channel at www.youtube.com/stew50smith to find over 120 exercise videos, swim technique videos, and even some of these workouts. You can also find all the videos in the easy-to-use free app Navy SEAL Exercises with Stew Smith, available on both Apple and Android devices.

For more guidance, you check out some of my other workout collections (listed at the end of this book).

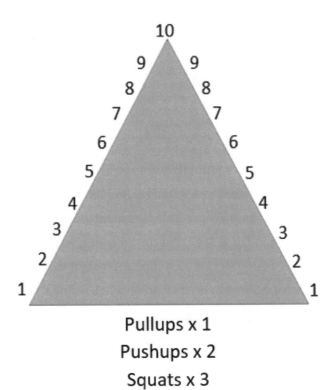

Pullups x 1
Pushups x 2
Squats x 3

If you take a look at the pyramid above, you will notice that it is numbered on both sides, going from 1–9 on the left with 10 on the top, then from 9–1 on the right. Each number represents a step in the pyramid. Your goal is to "climb" the pyramid all the way up and then all the way back down, so you can consider each step a "set" in your workout.

Here is how it works:

Starting at the bottom left of the pyramid, you will perform the lowest count "set" of your workout. For example: "Pull-ups x 1, push-ups x 2, sit-ups x 3." What this means is that at each set or "step" of the pyramid, you perform 1 pull-up for every step you are on, 2 push-ups for each step, and 3 sit-ups for each step. So at 6, you would be performing 6 pull-ups, 12 push-ups and 18 sit-ups.

You would then keep progressing until you either get to the top of the pyramid, or your max at failure. (Again, at step 10 you would be performing 10 pull-ups, 20 push-ups and 30 sit-ups.) Now, you start working your way back down the other side. The next set you do will be "repeating" step 9 on the way back down, completing 9 pull-ups, 18 push-ups and 27 sit-ups. Keep going until you've worked all the way back down to step 1.

This is what makes the pyramid such an effective workout for high volumes of repetitions. For example, were you to do pull-ups for each level of the above 1–10–1 pyramid, you would achieve 100 pull-ups. It also means pyramids are great as an "in-workout" assessment tool. Let's say you do the pyramid one day and fail at set 8, but the following week you fail at set 9 or 10. You can see your progress each time you repeat the workout, just as you can see increased weight on the barbell when lifting.

Performing Pyramid Workouts

Start from the bottom at set 1 and perform the listed exercises. For each set (or "step") of the pyramid, perform the same exercises again while increasing the number of reps by a multiple of the current step. For example, 1 push-up and 2 sit-ups on step 1 becomes 5 push-ups and 10 sit-ups on step 5. Continue until you reach the listed "top" of the pyramid, then repeat the previous steps in reverse order to "descend" the pyramid.

THE
WORKOUTS

Pyramid
Warmups

1
UPPER BODY WORKOUT
WARMUP

This warmup is perfect for 5–10 minutes prior to a bench press workout or high repetition calisthenics workout. Typically, anything after 10 reps in a pyramid becomes part of a workout, so there's no need to return in reverse order. Just stop at 5-10 and move onto your upper body push workout. (You can do the same thing with pull-ups.)

1–10 Ladder: Push-ups
Perform 1 push-up for each step of the ladder, starting from step 1. Progress from 1 to 10, jogging 25–50 meters (with dynamic stretches) at an easy pace between each set, for a total of 55 push-ups and 250–500 meters.

2
LOWER BODY WORKOUT WARMUP

You can do this warmup prior to leg day, regardless of whether the workout is a lift workout, run workout, or high repetition calisthenics workout. Remember, anything after 10 reps in a pyramid becomes part of a workout so there's no need to return in reverse order. Just stop at 5–10 and move on to your leg workout.

1–10 Ladder: Squats
Perform 1 squat for each step of the ladder, starting from step 1. Progress from 1 to 10, jogging 25–50 meters (with dynamic stretches) at an easy pace between each set, for a total of 55 squats and 250–500 meters.

3
FULL BODY WORKOUT WARMUP

Calling this a warmup is a little deceptive, as it can quickly turn into a workout depending on your fitness level. Can you do this one non-stop to level 10? Then this is a good warmup for you. If not, you might want to start with 1–5 and build up from there.

1–20 Ladder: Burpees

Perform 1 burpee for each step of the ladder, starting from step 1. Progress from 1 to 20, running 100 yards between each set, for a total of 210 squats and 2000 yard.

4
CARDIO WARMUP PYRAMID

1–10 Ladder: Cardio Warm-up

If you prefer your warmups to be more of a traditional cardio option, you can also pyramid each minute by increasing speed, resistance, or elevation, depending on the cardio machine, for 5–10 minutes. Increase speed by a mile/km per hour, increase resistance, or elevation by one level each minute for 5–10 minutes depending on your time to train and abilities.

Upper Body
Pyramids

5
THE #1 CLASSIC PT PYRAMID

This is *the* classic pyramid…albeit with a few upgrades. Note that many branches of service are getting rid of sit-ups and replacing them with plank poses or knee-ups in their fitness testing, so feel free to substitute as preferred. (However, many groups—including special ops—are still using sit-ups as part of their training/testing, so don't stop doing them just yet!)

1–10–1 Pyramid: Pull-ups/Push-ups/Sit-ups
Perform 1 pull-up, 2 push-ups and 3 sit-ups for each step of the pyramid. Continue to progress up the pyramid until you fail or reach 10 sets, then repeat in reverse order for a total of 100 pull-ups, 200 push-ups and 300 sit-ups.

6
MODIFIED CLASSIC PT PYRAMID: DIPS

The first of my twists on the classic pyramid formula, this version adds the option of dips, plank pose or knee-ups for additional triceps/shoulder burn. Try to do the same number of dips as you would push-ups. Note that you can also try this as a half-pyramid to start. Performing over 20 reps of knee-ups in a single set can be challenging, so try to mix things up with a variety of core exercises.

1–10–1 Pyramid: Pull-ups/Push-ups/Sit-ups/Dips

Perform 1 pull-up, 2 push-ups and 3 sit-ups (or 3 seconds plank or 3 knee-ups) and 2 dips for each step of the pyramid. Continue to progress up the pyramid until you fail or reach 10 sets, then repeat in reverse order for a total of 100 pull-ups, 200 push-ups, 300 sit-ups and 200 dips.

7
MODIFIED CLASSIC PT PYRAMID: RUNNING OPTION A

The classic 1–10–1 PT pyramid has 19 sets in it. This large number of sets makes any added running completely change the workout in multiple different ways. I've included several variations on this theme. Note: The distance run for each step of the pyramid is static, meaning it does not increase as you climb the pyramid. You'll run the same distance at step 9 that you ran at step 1, in this case 100 meters, for a total of 1900 meters by the end.

1–10–1 Pyramid: Pull-ups/Push-ups/Sit-ups

Perform 1 pull-up, 2 push-ups and 3 sit-ups for each step of the pyramid. In between each set, run 100 meters at sprint pace. Continue to progress up the pyramid until you fail or reach 10 sets, then repeat in reverse order for a total of 100 pull-ups, 200 push-ups, 300 sit-ups and 1900 meters.

8
MODIFIED CLASSIC PT PYRAMID: RUNNING OPTION B

This version of the classic PT pyramid calls for a greater distance than the previous option, and at goal mile pace. Note: The distance run for each step of the pyramid is static, meaning it does not increase as you climb the pyramid. You'll run the same distance at step 9 that you ran at step 1, in this case 400 meters, for a total of 7600 meters (or 4.75 miles) by the end.

1–10–1 Pyramid: Pull-ups/Push-ups/Sit-ups

Run 400 meters at goal mile pace, then perform 1 pull-up, 2 push-ups and 3 sit-ups for each step of the pyramid. In between each set, continue to run 400 meters at goal mile pace. Continue to progress up the pyramid until you fail or reach 10 sets, then repeat in reverse order for a total of 100 pull-ups, 200 push-ups, 300 sit-ups and 8000 meters.

9
MODIFIED CLASSIC PT PYRAMID: RUNNING OPTION C

This version again increases the distance run per set, but decreases the number of sets to every *other* interval. Note: The distance run for each step of the pyramid is static, meaning it does not increase as you climb the pyramid. You'll run the same distance at step 9 that you ran at step 1, in this case 800 meters, for a total of 8000 meters (or 5 miles) by the end.

1–10–1 Pyramid: Pull-ups/Push-ups/Sit-ups

Run 800 meters at goal mile pace, then perform 1 pull-up, 2 push-ups and 3 sit-ups for each step of the pyramid. In between every other set, continue to run 800 meters at goal mile pace. Continue to progress up the pyramid until you fail or reach 10 sets, then repeat in reverse order for a total of 100 pull-ups, 200 push-ups, 300 sit-ups and 8000 meters.

10
MODIFIED CLASSIC PT
PYRAMID: RUNNING OPTION D

This version keeps the same approximate running distance as the previous option, but increases the distance run per set while further decreases the number of running intervals. Here, you'll run 1 mile every 4–5 sets, for a total of 4–5 miles over the course of the workout.

1–10–1 Pyramid: Pull-ups/Push-ups/Sit-ups

Run 1 mile at goal mile pace, then perform 1 pull-up, 2 push-ups and 3 sit-ups for each step of the pyramid. Every 4–5 sets, continue to run 1 mile at goal mile pace. Continue to progress up the pyramid until you fail or reach 10 sets, then repeat in reverse order for a total of 100 pull-ups, 200 push-ups, 300 sit-ups and 4–5 miles.

11
MODIFIED CLASSIC PT PYRAMID: WEIGHTED

By using some form of added resistance, such as from a weight vest or TRX, you can either make the classic PT pyramid workout much easier or much tougher. The addition of the TRX in particular is helpful especially if you fail at pull-ups or want to make your push-ups tougher. Replace the pull-ups with TRX rows when you reach failure (to make them easier) or do atomic push-ups with the TRX to make the push-ups much harder.

1–10–1 Pyramid: Pull-ups/Push-ups/Sit-ups
Perform 1 pull-up (or TRX row), 2 push-ups (or TRX atomic push-ups) and 3 sit-ups for each step of the pyramid. Continue to progress up the pyramid until you fail or reach 10 sets, then repeat in reverse order for a total of 100 pull-ups (or TRX row), 200 push-ups (or TRX atomic push-ups) and 300 sit-ups.

12
PT PYRAMID MAX EFFORT WITH RUN WARMUP/COOLDOWN

This workout is best done outside in a space where you have access pull-up bar, or else on a field with plenty of room. For extra credit, try adding other forms of travel to make the workout tougher, such as fireman carries, bear crawls, crab walks, farmer walks, walking lunges, etc.

Warm-Up
Run 1.5 mile

1–15/20 Pyramid: Push-ups/Pull-ups
Perform 1 push-up and 1 pull-up for each step of the pyramid, alternating each with a 50 meter run. Progress from 1 to 10; if you fail at 10 sets or less, repeat in reverse order back down to 1. If you get above 10, keep going up the pyramid until you fail at any exercise; do not repeat in reverse order.

Run 50 meters

Cooldown
Run 1.5 mile

13
BURPEE LADDER

This workout makes use of a ladder (or half-pyramid), a format which follows the pyramid's rule of increasing reps each step, but which does not feature the descent back "down" the pyramid. The burpees (or 8-count bodybuilder push-ups, if your prefer) in this workout act as more of an active rest for the other max effort exercises (pull-ups, dips, abs) and vice versa. Try mixing this constant movement pyramid into your upper body circuit.

1–5 Ladder: Burpees

Jog 25 meters, then perform 1 burpee for each step of the ladder. Continue to progress up the ladder, jogging 25 meters between each step, for a total of 15 burpees. Use dynamic stretches in between intervals.

Pull-ups – max effort
Dips – max effort
Abs of choice – 50 reps OR plank pose – 1 minute

6–10 Ladder: Burpees

Run 25 meters, then perform 1 burpee for each step of the ladder, starting from step 6. Continue to progress up the ladder to step 10, running 25 meters between each step, for a total of 40 burpees.

Repeat 2 times
Pull-ups – max effort
Dips – 10–15 reps
Abs of choice – 50 reps

11–15 Ladder: Burpees

Run 25 meters, then perform 1 burpee for each step of the
ladder, starting from step 11. Continue to progress up
the ladder to step 15, running 25 meters between each
step, for a total of 65 burpees.

Repeat 3 times
Pull-ups – max effort
TRX push-ups OR regular push-ups – max effort
Abs of choice – 50 reps OR plank pose – 1 minute

16–20 Ladder: Burpees

Run 25 meters, then perform 1 burpee for each step of the
ladder, starting from step 16. Continue to progress up
the ladder to step 20, running 25 meters between each
step, for a total of 90 burpees.

14
THE 8-COUNT BODY BUILDER/ PULL-UP PYRAMID

For this pyramid, I invite you to get creative on your even sets and mix things up with alternate movements such as bear crawls, low crawls, fireman carries or body drags. Try not to repeat the same one too many times.

Warm-Up
Run 1 mile OR 10 minute bike

1–15/20 Pyramid: Pull-ups/Burpees
Perform 1 pull-up and 1 burpee for each step of the pyramid, alternating each with a 25 meter run. Progress from 1 to 10; if you fail at pull-ups in 10 sets or less, repeat in reverse order back down to 1. If you get above 10, keep going up the pyramid until you fail at any exercise; do not repeat in reverse order.

Cooldown
Run 2 miles cooldown

15
CLASSIC PT PYRAMID WARMUP WITH PT TEST MIX

1–5 Ladder: Pull-ups/Push-ups/Sit-ups
Perform 1 pull-up, 2 push-ups and 3 sit-ups for each step
of the ladder. Progress from 1 to 5. Perform dynamic
stretches for 25 meters after each set, such as butt
kickers, leg swings, side steps, etc.

Pull-ups – max
Push-ups – max 2 minutes
Sit-ups – 2 minutes

Run 1 mile

Repeat 2 times
Pull-ups – max
Push-ups – to failure, remain in plank for extra 1 minute
Sit-ups – max 1 minute
Run 1 mile

5–1 Ladder: Pull-ups/Push-ups/Sit-ups
Perform 1 pull-up, 2 push-ups and 3 sit-ups for each step
of the ladder, starting from step 5. Progress from 5 to 1.
Perform dynamic stretches for 25 meters after each set,
such as butt kickers, leg swings, side steps, etc.

16
RUN AND PT PYRAMID WARMUP WITH PST EVENTS

This workout focuses on improving on any weak areas you might have shown during your last PST. After completing the 1.5 mile timed run, choose ONE of the available options that best corresponds with your target event.

Warm-Up
Run 1 mile

1–10 Ladder: Pull-ups/Running/Push-ups
Perform 1 pull-up for each step of the pyramid, run 30 meters, then perform 1 push-up for each step of the pyramid. Progress from 1 to 10, then back down to 1, including a 30 meter run at each step for a total of 570 meters. Alternate runs with dynamic stretches as necessary.

500 yard swim OR bike 10 minutes
Push-ups – 2 minutes max reps
Sit-ups –2 minutes max reps
Pull-ups – max
1.5 mile timed run

Choose ONE of the following:

Repeat 4 times
Push-ups – 1 minute push-up test
Rest with sit-ups – 1 minute at goal pace
Pull-ups – 1 minute

Repeat 6 times
Run 400 meters at goal mile pace
Rest with 1 minute walk

Repeat 5 times
Swim 50 meters freestyle, fast
Swim 50 meters CSS at goal pace

17
PLUS DAY RUNS AND PULL-UPS

Warm-Up
Pull-ups – 2,4,6,8,10
Between each set of reps, stretch legs to prep for run

Repeat 3–4 times
Run 1 mile OR bike 7 minutes
Pull-ups – max
Pulldowns – 10 reps
Dumbbell Rows – 10 per arm

18
RUNNING AND PULL-UPS/ PUSH-UP PYRAMID

Warm-Up
Pull-ups – 2,4,6,8,10
Between each set of reps, do short 25–50 meter jogs with
   dynamic stretches to prep for run

Repeat 3–4 times
Run 1 mile
Pull-ups – max OR TRX rows/pulldowns if failure 5–10 reps
Push-ups – max
Sit-ups – 1 minute OR TRX atomic push-ups: try to double
   your pull-up reps each set
Ruck OR swim with fins – 30 minutes

19
BURPEE/PULL-UP PYRAMID: 1–10–1 CHALLENGE

For this pyramid challenge, you can replace the burpees with burpee push-ups or 8-count bodybuilder push-ups, if you're looking to change things up.

Warm-Up
Run 1.5 miles

1–10–1 Pyramid: Pull-ups/Burpees
Run 25–50 meters, then perform 1 pull-up and 1 burpee for each step of the pyramid. Progress from 1 to 10, then back down to 1, including a 25–50 meter run every interval for a total of 100 pull-ups/burpees and 475–950 meters.

Cooldown
Run 1.5 mile cooldown

20
BURPEE/PULL-UP LADDER: 1–20 CHALLENGE

Just as with the previous pyramid, you can replace the burpees with burpee push-ups or 8-count bodybuilder push-ups, if you're looking for greater variety. This works best if you have an outdoor pull-up bar or a pull-up bar in an open area (like a basketball court).

Warm-Up
Run 1.5 miles

1–20 Ladder: Pull-ups/Burpees
Perform 1 pull-up and 1 burpee for each step of the pyramid. Progress from 1 to 20, for a total of 210 pull-ups/burpees.

21
RUN AND PT CHALLENGE

Warm-Up
5 minutes jog

Pull-ups – 2,4,6,8,10
Perform 10 push-ups and 10 sit-ups in between each set of pull-ups, using a different grip for each set (wide, regular, reverse, close, commando or alternating grip)

22
100M BURPEE PYRAMID
+ PT PYRAMID

1–20+ Ladder: Burpees

Perform 1 burpee for each step in the ladder, then get up and run 100 yards. Keep going until you run out of time or energy, with a goal of 20 sets in 30–40 minutes.

1 mile timed run

1–10+ Ladder: Pull-ups/Dips/Sit-ups

Perform 1 pull-up, 2 dips and 5 sit-ups (or abs of choice) for each step of the ladder. How high can you go up the ladder pyramid until you fail at both pull-ups and dips? Shoot for 10+ sets.

Cooldown

1 mile run

23
PUSH-UP DOUBLED PYRAMID

Doubled Pyramid 2–10: Push-ups
Perform 2 push-ups for each step of the pyramid, progressing from 2, to 4, to 6, and so on. Progress to 10 reps on the fifth set, inserting 25 meter jogs/dynamic stretches in between each set.

Pull-ups – max effort
Dips – max effort
Abs of choice – 50 OR 1 minute plank pose

Doubled Pyramid 12–20: Push-ups
Perform 2 push-ups for each step of the pyramid, starting from 12. Progress to 20 reps on the fifth set, inserting 25 meter jogs/dynamic stretches in between each set.

Pull-ups – max effort
Overhead press – 10-15 OR hand stand push-ups – 10-15
Abs of choice – 50 OR 1 minute plank pose

Doubled Pyramid 22–30: Push-ups

Perform 2 push-ups for each step of the pyramid, starting from 22. Progress to 30 reps on the fifth set, inserting 100 meter runs in between each set.

Pull-ups – max effort
Dips – max effort
Plank pose – 1 minute

Cooldown

Run 2 miles OR swim 1000 meters

24
BURPEE PYRAMID MIX

Burpee or push-up pyramid workouts make for great upper body warm-ups...
until you reach set 10 in the pyramid. Anything after 10 reps of any exercise in
this "warm-up pyramid" becomes a significant part of the workout challenge.
Keep track of your number of pull-ups, dips and sit-ups in the final set for PT
purposes.

1–5 Ladder: Burpees

Perform 1 burpee for each step in the ladder, then get
up and jog 25–50 meters (with dynamic stretches).
Progress from 1 to 5, including a 25–50 meter jog at
each step for a total of 15 burpees and 125–250 meters.
Alternate runs with dynamic stretches as necessary.

Repeat 2 times

Pull-ups – max effort
Dips – max effort
Abs of choice – 50 OR 1 minute plank pose

6–10 Ladder: Burpees

Perform 1 burpee for each step in the ladder, then get up
and run 25 meters. Progress from 6 to 10, including a
25 meter run at each step for a total of 40 burpees and
125 meters.

Repeat 2 times
Pull-ups – max effort
Push press – 10
Abs of choice – 50
Bench press – 10

11–15 Ladder: Burpees/Push-ups
Perform 1 burpee (or push-up) for each step in the ladder, then get up and run 25 meters. Progress from 11 to 15, including a 25 meter run at each step for a total of 65 burpees and 125 meters.

Repeat 2 times
TRX rows – 10 OR pulldowns (heavy) – 10
Bench press – 10 OR TRX push-ups – max
1 minute plank pose OR TRX rollouts – 10

16–20 Ladder: Burpees/Push-ups
Perform 1 burpee (or push-up) for each step in the ladder, then get up and run 25 meters. Progress from 16 to 20, including a 25 meter run at each step for a total of 90 burpees and 125 meters.

Pull-ups – max effort
Dips – max effort
Sit-ups – 2 minutes

25
DEATH BY PUSH-UPS PYRAMID

1–20 Ladder: Death by Push-Ups

Hold a push-up position for 20 minutes. Each minute, add 1 push-up: 1 push-up the first minute, 2 push-ups the second minute, and so on, up to 20 push-ups during the final minute for a total of 210 push-ups. Your knees should not touch the ground throughout.

26
TRX PYRAMID

While the classic PT pyramid makes for a great workout when you first start doing it, after a while it makes for a better warm-up than an actual challenge. So. if you want a change of pace and a way to make a tough workout even tougher, try adding the TRX and replacing some of the standard exercises with these updated options. (You may want to limit the number of TRX rollouts and replace with an abs exercise of your choice or 30 seconds plank pose—particularly if you're new to the TRX.)

1–10–1 Pyramid: TRX Rows, Atomic Push-ups and Rollouts

Perform 1 TRX row, 2 TRX atomic push-ups and 3 TRX rollouts for each step of the pyramid. Progress from 1 to 10 (or until failure), then back down to 1.

27
PUSH FOCUS PYRAMID

This uses the classic pyramid repetition/set scheme but focuses on a single muscle group for the duration. I've included both a push-focused and pull-focused version of this concept. You may find that the push-ups are the hardest part of this workout, so if you need to adjust, change it to a x2 set multiplier.

Warm-Up
Jog 10 minutes, mixing in 5-10 push-ups every minute. Mix in some dynamic stretches and upper body stretches as needed.

1–10 Ladder: Push Exercises
Perform 2 bench presses, 2 dips and 2 military presses and 3 push-ups for each step of the ladder. Progress from 1 to 10, for a total of 110 bench presses, dips and military presses, and 165 push-ups.

28
PUSH FOCUS REVERSE PYRAMID

If you want to really up the ante from the previous Push Pyramid workout, try this one in reverse pyramid style (10–1) and make each set heavier, building up to a 1 repetition max (1RM). Though, with this level of volume, it'll be one very tired 1RM.

10–1 Reverse Ladder: Push Exercises

Perform 2 bench presses, 2 dips and 2 military presses and 3 push-ups for each step of the ladder, starting with 20 bench presses, 20 dips, 20 military presses and 30 push-ups at step 10. Progress from 10 to 1, for a total of 110 bench presses, dips and military presses, and 165 push-ups.

29
PULL FOCUS PYRAMID

For the pull focused pyramid, we select four pulling exercises that work the biceps, forearms, and latissimus dorsi (back muscles), which are mainly responsible for pulling away from the body (up, down, forward). You may find that the pulldowns are the hardest part of this workout. If you need to adjust, change it to a x2 set multiplier.

1–10 Ladder: Pull Exercises

Perform 1–2 pull-ups, 2 rows, 2 bicep curls and 3 pulldowns for each step of the ladder. Progress from 1 to 10, for a total of 55–110 pull-ups, 110 rows and bicep curls, and 165 pulldowns. Run for 5 minutes every 5 sets, or else run 20 minutes (or other cardio) at the end of the pyramid.

Swim 150 meters + 50 abs of choice – AMRAP in 30 minutes

30
PULL FOCUS REVERSE PYRAMID

If you want to really up the ante from the previous Pull Pyramid workout, try this one in reverse pyramid style (10–1) and make each set heavier, building up to a 1 repetition max (1RM). Though, with this level of volume, it'll be one very tired 1RM.

10–1 Reverse Ladder: Pull Exercises

Perform 1–2 pull-ups, 2 rows, 2 bicep curls and 3 pulldowns for each step of the ladder, starting with 20 pull-ups, 20 rows, 20 bicep curls and 30 pulldowns at step 10. Progress from 10 to 1, for a total of 55–110 pull-ups, 110 rows and bicep curls, and 165 pulldowns.

31
PULL-UPS/BURPEE RUN
PYRAMID WITH PT RESET

The pull-ups/burpee and run pyramid is a workout that will challenge your heart and lungs as well as your pushing, pulling, and grip muscles. You may find that, after a series of pull-ups and burpees, it takes about 2–3 minutes before you feel like you are running efficiently. This is common and very helpful when preparing your body for physical fitness tests. Prepare your body for quick lactate buffering with this workout and build a body that can crush PT/run fitness tests!

Warm-Up
5 minutes dynamic stretches

1–5 Pyramid: Pull-ups/Burpees
Perform 1 pull-up and 1 burpee for each step of the pyramid, starting from 1 and progressing to 5. Insert a short 25 meter run between each set of pull-ups/burpees for a total of 125 meters.

Run 1 mile
Reverse push-ups – 20
Birds – 20
Arm haulers – 20

6–10 Pyramid: Pull-ups/Burpees

Perform 1 pull-up and 1 burpee for each step of the pyramid, starting from 6 and progressing to 10. Insert a short 25 meter run between each set of pull-ups/burpees for a total of 125 meters.

Run 1 mile
Reverse push-ups – 20
Birds – 20
Arm haulers – 20

10–6/11–15 Pyramid: Pull-ups/Burpees

Perform 1 pull-up and 1 burpee for each step of the pyramid, starting from 10 and progressing down to 6 OR starting from 11 and progressing to 15, if you're looking for extra challenge. Insert a short 25 meter run between each set of pull-ups/burpees for a total of 125 meters.

Run 1 mile
Reverse push-ups – 20
Birds – 20
Arm haulers – 20

5–1/16–20 Pyramid: Pull-ups/Burpees

Perform 1 pull-up and 1 burpee for each step of the pyramid, starting from 5 and progressing down to 1 OR starting from 16 and progressing to 20, if you're looking for extra challenge. Insert a short 25 meter run between each set of pull-ups/burpees for a total of 125 meters.

Reverse push-ups – 20
Birds – 20
Arm haulers – 20

32
PT PYRAMID CHALLENGE: 1–15–1

This one is for those who are having an easy day with the standard 1–10–1 pyramid and are starting to work their way up to the 1–20 half-pyramid. This 1–15–1 will total 225 repetitions of any exercise included, which is 450 reps of any doubled exercise. That is *a lot* of volume. Can you handle it?

1–15–1 Pyramid: Pull-ups/Push-ups/Abs of choice

Perform 1 pull-up, 2 push-ups and 3 abs of choice exercises for each step of the pyramid. Progress from 1 to 15, then back down to 1. Use a variety of abs exercises to completely work your core, since you'll be getting 675 reps of any exercise you select.

33
PULL-UP PYRAMID
WITH ABS WORK

1–10 Pyramid: Pull-ups

Perform 1 pull-up for each step of the pyramid, progressing from 1 to 10 for a total of 55 pull-ups.

Crunches OR Reverse crunches – 25
Sit-ups – 25 OR 30 seconds plank pose
Hanging Knee-ups – 10

10–1 Pyramid: Reverse Grip Pull-ups

Perform 1 reverse grip pull-up for each step of the pyramid, starting with 10 reps, progressing from 10 to 1 for a total of 55 pull-ups.

34
WEIGHTED PUSH AND PULL PYRAMID

1–10 Ladder: Push-ups/Pull-ups
Perform 1 push-up and 1 pull-up for each step in the
   ladder, then get up and run 25 meters. Progress from
   1 to 10, running 25 meters between each step. Stretch
   as needed.

Bench press (heavy weight) – 5 rep max
Pulldowns (heavy weight) – 5 rep max

Bench press – 4,4,3,3,2,2,1,1 reps, increase weight each set
Pulldowns – 4,4,3,3,2,2,1,1 reps, increase weight each set

Swimmers – 1 minute
Plank pose – 1 minute
Reverse push-ups – 25
Birds – 25
Arm haulers – 25
Run 1.5–3 miles timed
Swim 500 meters warm-up pace

Repeat 10 times
Swim freestyle – 50 meters, fast
Swim CSS – 50 meters goal pace

35
REVERSE PUSH-UPS/ FLUTTERKICKS PYRAMID

25–1 Reverse Ladder: Push-ups/Flutterkicks

Perform 1 push-up and 1 flutterkick for each step of the pyramid, beginning at step 25 with 25 push-ups and 25 flutterkicks. Progress from step 25 to step 1, for a total of 325 push-ups and flutterkicks. With each set of flutterkicks, alternate your positioning. On odd-numbered sets of flutterkicks, perform the movement on your back; on even-numbered sets, perform the movement on your belly.

36
PULL-UPS/BURPEE TIMED PYRAMID

Timed Ladder: Pull-ups/Burpees

Run 50 meters, then perform 1 burpee and 1 pull-up for each step of the ladder. Continue to progress up the pyramid, running 50 meters between each step, for a total time of 30 minutes. How high can you get?

1–10 Ladder: Swimming PT

Perform 2 push-ups and 3 abs of choice for each step of the ladder, starting from step 1. Progress from 1 to 10, swimming 100 meters in between every set for a total of 110 push-ups, 165 abs of choice, and 1000 meters swimming.

Lower Body
Pyramids

37
TRACK/RUN AND LEG PT PYRAMID

Warm-Up
1 mile warmup jog or 5 minutes bike/stretch
1 mile timed run

Repeat 10 times
400 meters at goal mile pace
Rest with pyramid leg/ab exercises of your choice – 10 sets

Options for 400m
If you want some jog/sprint combos, try jogging the corners of the track and sprinting the straights, alternating 100 meters for each pace.

Cooldown
5 sets of 100 meters swims at goal pace
Rest 30 seconds
10 sets of 50 meters at goal pace for 500 meters

38
LEG DAY WITH CARDIO INTERVALS

1–20 Ladder: 25m Run/Burpees

Run 25 meters, then perform 1 burpee for each step of the ladder. Continue to progress up the ladder, running 25 meters between each step, for a total of 210 burpees. You can also do dynamic stretches in between burpee sets (butt kickers, leg swings, other stretches).

1–10 Ladder: Burpee/Stair Climb

Repeat the above pyramid, replacing the 25 meter runs with runs up and down a flight of steps in between each set, until you reach 10 sets.

Cooldown

Swim 20–30 minutes with fins OR complete a bike pyramid (below)

Bike Pyramid

Bike for 10–15 minutes, making each minute harder by adding a level of resistance (or two), then repeat in reverse order. Keep your RPMs at 70–90.

39
AIR BURPEE PYRAMID

1–10 Ladder: 25m Run/Burpees

Run 25 meters, then perform 1 burpee for each step of the ladder. Continue to progress up the ladder, running 25 meters between each step, for a total of 55 burpees.

1–10 Ladder: Burpee/Weighted Stair Climb

Repeat the above pyramid, replacing the 25 meter runs with runs up and down a flight of steps in between each set while wearing a weighted vest of about 30 pounds, or else while carrying dumbbells. Complete one up/down set of stair climbs, then perform 1 burpee for each step of the ladder, for a total of 55 burpees. Stretch when needed.

40
BURPEE/STAIR CLIMB PYRAMID

1–10–1 Pyramid: Burpee/Stair Climb

Climb up and down a set of stairs, then perform 1 burpee for each step in the pyramid. Continue up to 10 burpees, then repeat in reverse order for a total of 100 burpees and 19 up/down sets of stair climbs.

41
MILITARY LEG DAY

1–20 Ladder: Burpees/100m

Perform 1 burpee for each step of the ladder, then run 100 meters. Continue to progress up the ladder, running 100 meters after each increasing number of burpees, for a total of 210 burpees. Optionally, after each fifth set of burpees, instead of running 100 meters you can grab a partner of like weight and fireman carry them 50 meters, before changing with your partner to be carried a further 50 meters.

Burpee/Run

Run for 20 minutes. Every 5 minutes, stop and perform:
Burpees – 10–20 reps
Lunges – 10 per leg

Military PT Test

Choose one of the following:
Navy/Air Force – Run 1.5 miles, timed
Army – Run 2 miles, timed
USMC – Run 3 miles, timed

Choose 1 of the following:

Navy/Air Force/USMC RECON – Swim 500 meters warm-up with no fins, then swim 1000 meters with fins
Army/USMC – Ruck 30 minutes for max distance

42
RUN AND LEG PT

Warm-Up
5 minute run or bike

Track/Field Workout
Run 100 meters / 20 burpees and 10 lunges per leg
Run 200 meters / 20 burpees and 10 lunges per leg
Run 300 meters / 20 burpees and 10 lunges per leg
Run 400 meters / 20 burpees and 10 lunges per leg
Run 300 meters / 20 burpees and 10 lunges per leg
Run 200 meters / 20 burpees and 10 lunges per leg
Run 100 meters / 20 burpees and 10 lunges per leg

43
RUN AND LEG PT PYRAMID

Warm-Up
Jog 1 mile, then stretch

Repeat 2 times
Run 400 meters, fast
40 burpees
Run 300 meters, fast
30 burpees
Run 200 meters, fast
20 lunges per leg
Run 100 meters, fast
10 lunges per leg

Full Body Calisthenics/ Resistance & Cardio Pyramids

44
PULL-UP/DEAD LIFT RUN DAY

1–10 Pyramid: Pull-up/Deadlift

Perform 1 pull-up and 10 deadlifts (start with moderately
    light weight, but know that you will have to make
    it heavier it as you go). For each step in the ladder,
    increase the number of pull-ups by 1 and decrease
    the number of deadlifts by 1. Keep going up the pull-
    up pyramid and down the deadlift until you reach 10
    pull-ups and 1 deadlift. If you fail at pull-ups at any
    point, repeat in reverse order (lightening the deadlifts if
    needed). Repeat for 25 minutes total time.

Cooldown

Run or swim with fins – 25 minutes for max distance

45
UPPER BODY PT PYRAMID

1–10–1 Pyramid: Pull-ups/TRX Push-ups/ Kettlebell Swing

Perform 1 pull-up, 2 TRX push-ups and 3 kettlebell swings for each step of the pyramid. Continue to progress up the pyramid, running for 1 mile at fast pace in between every fifth set. Keep going until you fail or reach 10 sets, then repeat in reverse order for a total of 100 pull-ups, 200 TRX push-ups and 300 kettlebell swings. (If you need to resort to regular push-ups to complete the workout, then do so.)

Cooldown

500 meter timed swim – any stroke
Swim –10 minutes
Tread water (with or without hands) – 10 minutes
Dynamic stretches in chest deep water – 10 minutes

46
PT PYRAMID 1RM LIFTS

Here's a new twist to the PT pyramid. You'll be going UP the pyramid until you fail at calisthenics, while increasing the weight for your lifts as you decrease the number of reps.

1–10–1 Pyramid: Modified PT

Perform 1–2 pull-ups, 2–3 push-ups, 2–3 burpees, 1–2 dips and 3 abs of choice for each step of the pyramid. Continue to progress up the pyramid until you fail or reach 10 sets, then repeat in reverse order for a max total of 100–200 pull-ups, 200–300 push-ups, 200–300 burpees, 100–200 dips and 300 abs of choice.

Once the above is completed (or failure is reached), perform the following:

Lift Circuit

Each one of these exercises is performed in a circuit fashion: 5 sets each, starting at 10 reps of each exercise and decreasing rep count by 2 with each new set while increasing the weight used.

Pulldowns
Bench press
Leg press/deadlift OR weighted burpees
Bicep/military press
Plank pose – 1 minute

Break things down so your first set is 10 reps of each of the exercises, then rest in plank pose for 1 minute and take a water break. Repeat that sequence of exercises, plank pose and water break for each successive set. It is up to you and your abilities whether to make each set heavier or not.

47
MURPH SANDBAG PYRAMID

This pyramid is a mix of the Murph workout (100 pull-ups, 200 push-ups, 300 burpees) but with added sandbag exercises that are used in various log PT workouts featured in military selection programs.

1–10–1 Pyramid: Classic PT

Perform 1 pull-up, 2 sandbag push presses and 3 sandbag burpees for each step of the pyramid. Continue to progress up the pyramid until you fail or reach 10 sets, then repeat in reverse order for a total of 100 pull-ups, 200 sandbag push presses and 300 sandbag burpees.

48
MURPH PT PYRAMID WITH 1 MILE RUNS

In between each step of the pyramid, run 1 mile

1–5 Ladder: Pull-ups/Push-ups/Burpees
Perform 1 pull-up, 2 push-ups and 3 burpees for each step of the pyramid. Continue to progress up the pyramid, doing dynamic stretches for 25 meters after each set, for a total of 15 pull-ups, 30 push-ups and 45 burpees.

6–10 Ladder: Pull-ups/Push-ups/Burpees
Continue the above ladder, starting at step 6 of the pyramid, for an additional total of 40 pull-ups, 80 push-ups and 120 burpees.

10–6 Ladder: Pull-ups/Push-ups/Burpees
Repeat the previous ladder in reverse, starting at step 10 of the pyramid and progressing down to step 6, for an additional total of 40 pull-ups, 80 push-ups and 120 burpees.

1–5 Ladder: Pull-ups/Push-ups/Burpees
Repeat the first ladder in reverse, starting at step 5 of the pyramid and progressing down to step 1, for an additional total of 15 pull-ups, 30 push-ups and 45 burpees.

[Continued on next page]

Cooldown
Run 1 mile
Jog or bike 10 minutes, then stretch

49
FULL BODY PT 1–20 PYRAMID

Warm-Up
Run 5 minutes

1–20 Ladder: 25m Run/Push-ups/Burpee
Perform 1 push-up and 1 burpee for each step of the ladder. Continue to progress up the ladder, running 25 meters between each step, for a total of 210 push-ups and 210 burpees. After every fifth set, perform max dips and pull-ups.

Ladder Run
Run 2400 meters – goal pace (1.5 miles)
Run 1600 meters – goal pace (1 mile)
Run 800 meters – goal pace (½-mile)

50
PULL-UP HALF PYRAMID: FIVE GRIPS

Perform 5 sets of the following:
Pull-ups – 2,4,6,8,10
Change grips with each set: regular grip, reverse grip, close grip, wide grip, commando grip
Rest with 1 minute sit-ups/plank pose or other core exercise, as needed

Ladder: Swimming
Swim 10 laps – CSS timed
Swim 8 laps – Freestyle at 8–10 strokes per breath
Swim 6 laps – CSS timed
Swim 4 laps – Freestyle at 4–6 strokes per breath
Swim 2 laps – Over/under (1 length underwater, 1 length freestyle)

51
5-REP PYRAMID

Warm-Up
Run 1 mile/stretch

1–10 Ladder: 5-Rep Push-ups
Perform 5 push-ups for each step of the pyramid. Continue to progress up the pyramid until you fail or reach 10 sets, for a total of 275 push-ups. In between each set, hold push-up/plank position for 15 seconds, then perform the following:
Sit-ups – 20
Flutterkicks – 25 (four count)
Burpees – 20

52
1–10–1 CARDIO PYRAMID

1–10 Ladder: Burpee/Push-ups/Run
Perform 1 burpee, 1 push-ups and run 25 burpees for each step of the pyramid. Continue to progress up the pyramid, increasing the number of burpees and push-ups by 1 for each step, until you fail or reach 10 sets for a total of 55 burpees, 55 push-ups and 250 meters.

1–10 Ladder: Pull-ups/Push-ups/TRX Rollouts
Perform 1 pull-up, 2 push-ups (or max TRX push-ups), and 1 TRX rollout (or 5 seconds plank pose) for each step of the ladder. Continue to progress up the ladder, bear crawling for 25 meters between each step, for a total of 55 pull-ups, 110 push-ups and 55 TRX rollouts.

10–1 Reverse Ladder: Dips/Burpees/Sit-ups
Perform 1 dip, 2 burpees (while shoulder-carrying a sandbag or backpack), and 3 sit-ups for each step of the ladder, starting at step 10. Continue to progress down the ladder, bear crawling for 25 meters between each step, for a total of 55 dips, 110 burpees and 165 sit-ups.

Cooldown
Run 2 miles OR swim 1000 meters

53
BURPEES SUPERSET PYRAMID

Warm-Up
5 minutes jog

Repeat 3 times
1–10 Burpee Ladder - Start at 1 burpee and run 100 meters
    in between each step of the ladder
Pull-ups – max
Dips – max
Burpees – 25
Abs of choice – 50 OR 1 minute plank pose

Cooldown
1–2 mile run AND/OR 500–1000 meters swim

54
10 REP/SET PT PYRAMID

Warm-Up
Run 1 mile/stretch
Push-ups – 5 sets of 10 reps, increasing rep count by 10
    with each set for a total of 150 reps

In between each push-up set above, do the following:
Stay in push-up or plank position for 15 seconds, then roll
    over and do:
Pull-ups – max reps
Sit-ups – 40–50 reps in 1 minute
Flutterkicks – 25 reps (four count)
Then, stand up and do:
Burpees – 30

55
BURPEE PYRAMID WITH RUN AND STAIR CRAWLS

1–5 Pyramid: Burpees/30m Runs

Perform 1 burpee for each step of the ladder, then run 30 meters. Continue to progress up the ladder, running 30 meters between each step, for a total of 15 burpees and 150 meters.

Dips – max reps
Pull-ups – max reps
Stair crawls (down/up or bear crawl) – 50 meters

6–10 Pyramid: Burpees/30m Runs

Perform 1 burpee for each step of the ladder, starting from step 6, then run 30 meters. Continue to progress up the ladder, running 30 meters between each step, for a total of 40 burpees and 150 meters.

Dips – max reps
Pull-ups – max reps
Stair crawls (down/up or bear crawl) – 50 meters

[Continued on next page]

10–6 Pyramid: Burpees/30m Runs

Perform 1 burpee for each step of the ladder, starting from
step 10, then run 30 meters. Continue to progress down
the ladder, running 30 meters between each step, for a
total of 40 burpees and 150 meters. Alternatively, you
can continue up the ladder, starting from step 11 and
finishing at step 15 for a more challenging workout.

Dips – max reps
Pull-ups – max reps
Stair crawls (down/up or bear crawl) – 50 meters

5–1 Pyramid: Burpees/30m Runs

Perform 1 burpee for each step of the ladder, starting from
step 5, then run 30 meters. Continue to progress down
the ladder, running 30 meters between each step, for a
total of 15 burpees and 150 meters. Alternatively, you
can continue up the ladder, starting from step 16 and
finishing at step 20 for a more challenging workout.

Dips – max reps
Pull-ups – max reps
Stair crawls (down/up or bear crawl) – 50 meters

Cooldown

Run 2 miles OR swim 1000 meters

56
THE HUNDREDS PYRAMID WORKOUT

1–10 Ladder: Burpees/50m Run
Perform 1 burpee for each step of the ladder, then run 50 meters. Continue to progress up the ladder, running 50 meters between each step, for a total of 55 burpees.

Stair crawl (up/down or bear crawl) – 50 meters
The following can be performed any way you want, provided you hit the total rep count:
100 pull exercises (pull-ups, downs, rows, etc.)
200 push exercises
300 burpees (no weights)
400 abs of choice
500 seconds plank pose

You can do the above repetition in circuit max rep fashion or pick 2–3 exercises (resting with core work) and accumulate the above reps in as few sets as possible.

9–1 Ladder: Burpees/50m Run
Perform 1 burpee for each step of the ladder, starting from step 9, then run 50 meters. Continue to progress down the ladder, running 50 meters between each step, for a total of 45 burpees.

57
HUNDREDS WORKOUT: 1–10–1 STYLE

1–10 Ladder: Burpees/50m Run

Perform 1 burpee for each step of the ladder, then run 50 meters. Continue to progress up the ladder, running 50 meters between each step, for a total of 55 burpees.

1–10–1 Pyramid: Pull-up/Push-up/Burpees/Abs of choice/Plank Pose

Perform 1 pull-up, 2 push-ups, 3 burpees, 4 abs of choice and 5 seconds plank pose for each step of the pyramid. Continue to progress up the pyramid until you reach 10 sets, then repeat in reverse order for a total of 100 pull-ups, 200 push-ups, 300 burpees, 400 hundred abs of choice, and 500 seconds plank pose.

9–1 Ladder: Burpees/50m Run

Perform 1 burpee for each step of the ladder, starting from step 9, then run 50 meters. Continue to progress down the ladder, running 50 meters between each step, for a total of 45 burpees.

58
HARD REVERSE PYRAMID

20–16 Ladder: Push-ups/Sit-ups/Arm Haulers
Perform 1 push up, 1 sit-up and 1 arm hauler for each step
of the ladder, starting at step 20, and work your way
down to step 16 for a total of 90 reps of each exercise.

Pull-ups – max reps
Dips – max reps

15–11 Ladder: Pull-ups/Push-ups/Sit-ups
Perform 1 pull-up, 1 push-up and 1 sit-up for each step of
the ladder, starting at step 15, and work your way down
to step 11 for a total of 65 reps of each exercise.

Flutterkicks (non stop) – 100 reps

10–6 Ladder: Pull-ups/Bench Press/Push Press
Perform 1 pull-up, 1 bench press and 1 push press for
each step of the ladder, starting at step 10, and work
your way down to step 6 for a total of 40 reps of each
exercise. Target 50% max rep up to body weight for the
push presses.

Run 1 mile or bike 10 minutes
5–1 Ladder: Pull-ups/Push Press/Kettlebell Clean and Press

[Continued on next page]

Perform 1 pull-up, 1 push press and 1 kettlebell clean and press for each step of the ladder, starting at step 5, and work your way down to step 1 for a total of 15 reps of each exercise.

59
5-MINUTE PYRAMIDS

5 minutes bike or elliptical Tabata interval: 20 seconds
fast/10 seconds easy
Increase level of resistance by 2 levels each minute for
5 minutes

5-Minute Pull-ups Pyramid
How high can you get up a pyramid of pull-ups in
5 minutes?

5-Minute Push-up/Plank Pose Pyramid
Stay in push-up position and perform a pyramid for the
listed exercises for as long as you can. Rest in the up
push-up position or plank pose.

**5-Minute Kettlebell Swings/Snatches/Clean
Press Pyramid**
Keep the kettlebell moving the entire time. Change arms
or use both arms, increasing up the pyramid non-stop.
Rest in rack position.

5 minutes walking lunges
Carry 25 pounds overhead for static press. Rest the weight
on your head if you must (best weight is a sandbag).
Keep doing walking lunges for 5 minutes non-stop.

[Continued on next page]

5 minutes Flutterkicks
No placing feet on floor. Keep moving your legs in the air for 5 minutes.

30 minutes run – max distance
30 minutes swim or ruck – max distance

60
X10 PYRAMID WARM-UP

x10 Pyramid: Push-Ups/Burpees

Perform 10 push-ups and 10 Burpees for each step of
the pyramid, then jog 200 meters. Continue to step 5,
jogging 200 meters in between each step, for a total of
150 push-ups, 150 burpees and 1000 meters.

Repeat 5 times

Pull-ups – 2,4,5,8,10

Each round, use a different grip for five total grips. When
you need a rest, do 20 burpees/20 push-ups or run
200 meters.

Cooldown

Run, swim or bike – 20 minutes (10 minutes easy, 10
minutes fast)

61
REVERSE X10 PYRAMID

x10 Pyramid: Push-Ups/Burpees
Perform 10 push-ups and 10 Burpees for each step of the pyramid, starting from step 5, then jog 200 meters. Progress down to step 1, jogging 200 meters in between each step, for a total of 150 push-ups, 150 burpees and 1000 meters.

Repeat 5 times
Pull-ups – max reps
Push Press – 20 reps
Burpees – 20 reps
Run 400 meters at goal mile pace (for timed runs)

Cooldown
Run, swim, or bike – 15 minutes

62
PARTNERED PUSH-UPS/
BURPEE LADDER

1–10 Ladder: Push-ups/Burpees

Run 25 meters, then perform 1 push-up and 1 burpee for each step of the ladder, starting from step 1. Progress from 1 to 10, running 25 meters in between every set, for a total of 110 push-ups, 110 burpees and 250 meters.

Have a partner hold plank pose for the amount of time it takes to complete the above ladder.

11–15 Ladder: Burpees

Run 25–50 meters, then perform 1 burpee for each step of the ladder, starting from step 11 and progressing to step 15. Run 25–50 meters in between every set, for a total of 65 burpees and 125–250 meters.

Have a partner walk up/down stairs with weight in hand for the amount of time it takes to complete the above ladder.

[Continued on next page]

16–20 Ladder: Burpees

Run 25–50 meters, then perform 1 burpee for each step of
the ladder, starting from step 16 and progressing to step
20. Run 25–50 meters in between every set, for a total
of 90 burpees and 125–250 meters.

Have a partner perform walking lunges for the amount of
time it takes to complete the above ladder.

63
FULL BODY X10 PYRAMID

Warm-Up
Run 1 mile, easy

1–4 x10 Pyramid: Push Press/Push-Ups/Sit-ups/ Burpees/Kettlebell Swings/Flutterkicks
Perform 10 push presses (40 pounds), 10 non-stop push-ups, 10 sit-ups (40 pounds), 10 burpees (40 pounds), 10 kettlebell swings and 10 flutterkicks for each step of the pyramid, starting from step 1, jogging 100 meters between each set. Progress to step 4, jogging 100 meters in between each step, for a total of 100 reps of each exercise and 400 meters. In addition, between each completed step of all listed exercises, perform one of the distance events listed below.

Distance Events
Bear Crawl – 100 meters/run 100 meters
Lunges – 100 meters (overhead carry, 40 pounds)/run 100 meters
Burpee Jumps – 100 meters/run 100 meters
Farmer Walk – 100 meters (40 pounds in each hand)/run 100 meters
Fireman Carry – 100 meters/run 100 meters
Sled or Prowler Push/Tow – 100 meters/run 100 meters

Cooldown
Run 1 mile easy

64
WEIGHTED CALISTHENICS/ CRAWLS PYRAMID

1–10–1 Pyramid: Weighted Pull-ups/Bench Press/Abs of Choice/Dips/Military Press

Perform 1 weighted pull-up (20–45 pounds), 2 bodyweight bench presses (or TRX push-ups), 3 abs of choice, 2 dips, and 2 military presses for each step of the pyramid. Continue to progress up the pyramid until you fail or reach 10 sets, then repeat in reverse order for a total of 100 weighted pull-ups, 200 bodyweight bench presses, 300 abs of choice, 200 dips, and 200 military presses. In between each step, run 200 meters. In between every fifth step, instead of running 200 meters, bear crawl for 100 meters.

65
PULL-UP, RUN, AND RUCK PYRAMID

Warm-Up
¼-mile jog OR 5 minute bike to stretch legs

3 mile ruck with 40–50 pounds weight

1–5 Ladder: Pull-ups
Perform 2 pull-ups for each step of the ladder, for each
of the following grips: regular, reverse, close, wide.
Continue to progress up the ladder until you reach 5
sets, for a total of 30 pull-ups per grip, or 120 total pull-
ups. Rest 20 seconds in plank pose between pull-up
sets for 8 minutes of plank pose total.

Repeat 8 times
400 meter repeats at goal mile pace
Burpees – 20 (perform during even sets)
Lunges – 10 per leg (perform during odd sets)
Consider adding weight to the lunges and burpees by
adding rucking to the calisthenics

Cooldown
5 minutes easy reverse bike pyramid or jog

66
WEIGHT-MODIFIED CLASSIC PYRAMID

1–10 Ladder: Pull-ups/Push-ups/Abs of Choice/Dips
Perform 1 pull-up, 2 push-ups, 3 abs of choice and 2 dips for each step of the pyramid. Continue to progress up the pyramid until you reach step 10, for a total of 55 pull-ups, 110 push-ups, 165 abs of choice and 110 dips. For added challenge, mix in some dynamic stretches in between sets, or add in a ½-mile run every fifth set.

1–10–1 Pyramid: Pull-ups/Pulldowns/Push-ups/Abs of choice/Dips
Perform 1 pull-up, 1 pulldown, 2 push-ups, 3 abs of choice and 2 dips for each step of the pyramid. Continue to progress up the pyramid until you fail or reach 10 sets. For the reverse order, add weights to each exercise, making them heavier as possible as you progress down the pyramid. This will result in a grand total of 100 pull-ups, 100 pulldowns, 200 push-ups, 300 abs of choice and 200 dips, half of which are weighted, half unweighted. Every fifth set, run 400 meters at goal mile pace.

67
FULL BODY PYRAMID

1–10–1 Pyramid: Full Body

Perform 1 pull-up, 3 push-ups, 2 push presses, 2 kettlebell swings and 2 burpees for each step of the pyramid. Continue to progress up the pyramid until you fail or reach 10 sets, then repeat in reverse order for a total of 100 pull-ups, 300 push-ups, 200 push presses, 200 kettlebell swings, and 200 burpees. Run 1 mile after every fifth set.

68
FULL BODY REVERSE PYRAMID

Warm-Up
Jog 5 minutes OR 1–10 burpee/push-up ladder with 25
   meter jogs between steps

Bench Press – 5 reps
Pulldowns – 5 reps
Deadlift – 5 reps

Reverse 20–16 Pyramid: Full Body
Perform 1 pull-up, abs of choice or push-up for each step of
   the pyramid, starting at step 20. Progress down to step
   16, running 25 meters between each step, for a total of
   90 exercises and 100 meters.

Bench Press – 5 reps
Hang Clean – 5 reps

Reverse 15–11 Pyramid: Full Body
Perform 1 pull-up, TRX rollout, kettlebell swing or 30
   seconds of plank pose for each step of the pyramid,
   starting at step 15. Progress down to step 11, running
   25 meters between each step, for a total of 65 exercises
   and 100 meters.

Bench Press – 5 reps
Push Press – 5-10 reps

Reverse 10–6 Pyramid: Full Body

Perform 1 pull-up, weighted burpee, TRX rollout, or 30 seconds of plank pose for each step of the pyramid, starting at step 10. Progress down to step 6, running 25 meters between each step, for a total of 40 exercises and 100 meters.

Reverse 5–1 Pyramid: Full Body

Perform 1 pull-up, bench press or deadlift for each step of the pyramid, starting at step 5. Progress down to step 1, running 25 meters between each step, for a total of 15 exercises and 100 meters. Use moderately heavier weight for each set of lifts, but avoid a 1-rep max level of weight.

Cooldown

2 mile run – easy pace
Swim 500 meters at warm-up pace, any stroke
Swim 300 meters at goal pace – 5 sets
Rest with 2 minutes plank pose, then swim 500 meters with fins

69
REVERSE PYRAMID WITH WEIGHTS/CALISTHENICS

This workout requires doing 20 reps of each exercise listed in a circuit: 19 reps, 18 reps, and so on. Run for 5 minutes every fifth set of this workout. Each cycle changes the exercises except for Pull-Ups which total 210 reps in this workout routine.

Reverse 20–16 Pyramid: Full Body

Perform 1 pull-up, 1 push-up and 1 sit-up for each step of the pyramid, starting at step 20. Progress down to step 16 for a total of 90 pull-ups, 90 push-ups and 90 sit-ups.

Run 5 minutes

Reverse 15–11 Pyramid: Full Body

Perform 1 pull-up, 1 bench press and 1 abs of choice for each step of the pyramid, starting at step 15. Progress down to step 11, for a total of 65 pull-ups, 65 bench presses, and 65 abs of choice.

Run 5 minutes

Reverse 10–6 Pyramid: Full Body

Perform 1 pull-up, 1 bench press and 1 weighted burpee for each step of the pyramid, starting at step 10. Progress down to step 6, for a total of 40 pull-ups, 40 bench presses and 40 weighted burpees.

Run 5 minutes

Reverse 5–1 Pyramid: Full Body

Perform 1 bench press, 1 deadlift and 1 weighted pull-up for each step of the pyramid, starting at step 5. Progress down to step 1, for a total of 15 bench presses, 15 deadlifts and 15 weighted pull-ups.

Cooldown

Swim 45 minutes or another non-impact cardio event of your choice

70
FULL BODY LADDER WITH LIFTS

1–15 Ladder: 25m Run/Push-Ups/Burpees
Run 25 meters, then perform 1 push-up and 1 burpee for
each step of the ladder. Continue to progress up the
ladder to step 15, running 25 meters between each step,
for a total of 120 push-ups, 120 burpees and 350 meters.

After every fifth set in the above ladder, do maximum effort
reps of the following exercises:
Bench Press – 10 reps
Pull-ups – max reps
Dips – max reps
Deadlift – 5 reps OR Leg Press – 10 reps

71
REVERSE PYRAMID:
MAX OUT WORKOUT

Max out on the following exercises within a 2 minute
    time limit, or until failure:
Pull-ups
Push-ups
Burpees
Sit-ups (or other abs of choice)

For the second set, max out again, but strive for the
    following goals:
Pull-ups – -2 from set 1 max
Push-ups – -10 from set 1 max
Burpees – -4 from set 1 max
Sit-ups – 2 minute goal pace

For the third set, max out again, but strive for the
    following goals:
Pull-ups – -4 from set 1 max
Push-ups – -20 from set 1 max
Burpees – -8 from set 1 max
Sit-ups – 2 minute goal pace

[Continued on next page]

For the fourth set, max out again, but strive for the
   following goals:
Pull-ups – -6 from set 1 max
Push-ups – -30 from set 1 max
Burpees – -12 from set 1 max
Sit-ups – 2 minute goal pace

For the fifth set, max out again, but strive for the
   following goals:
Pull-ups – -8 from set 1 max
Push-ups – -40 from set 1 max
Burpees – -16 from set 1 max
Sit-ups – 2 minute goal pace

Cardio
Pyramids

72
SWIMMING FOR DISTANCE PYRAMID

1–10–1 Swimming Pyramid: 100 Laps
Swim one 50 meter lap for each step in the pyramid,
    starting at step 1. Continue to progress up the pyramid
    until you reach 10 laps, then repeat in reverse order for
    a total of 100 laps or 5000 meters.

73
TIMED SWIM PYRAMID

1–10–1 Swimming Pyramid: 100 Laps
Swim one 50 meter lap for each step in the pyramid, starting at step 1. Continue to progress up the pyramid until you reach 10 laps, then repeat in reverse order for a total of 100 laps or 5000 meters. For each lap, focus on goal pace. If you can complete a 50 meter lap on a 1 minute interval, you'll complete this workout in 100 minutes. Your available time to rest between sets will be whatever the difference is between your goal pace and your lap time.

74
REVERSE SWIM LADDER FOR DISTANCE

Reverse Ladder: 100m Swim

Swim 100 meters for each step of the pyramid, starting with step 5. Progress down the ladder to step 1, for a total of 1500 meters. Rest as needed in between sets, making sure to focus on goal pace. Once you can complete this workout easily, incorporate the use of fins.

75
BIKE PYRAMID WORKOUT

1–15–1 Pyramid: Resistance Biking

Bike (on a stationary bike) for 1 minute at a starting resistance level. This is step 1 of the pyramid. After each minute/step, increase the resistance by 1–2 levels, to a max resistance at 15 minutes in (step 15). Then, repeat in reverse order for a total of 29 minutes. Try to keep the RPM of the stationary bike above 70rpm at a minimum. Once you are unable to maintain 70rpm, start to reduce the resistance in reverse order each minute.

76
ELLIPTICAL PYRAMID
WORKOUT

1–15–1 Pyramid: Resistance Elliptical

Workout on the elliptical for 1 minute at a starting
resistance level. This is step 1 of the pyramid. After
each minute/step, increase the resistance by 1–2 levels,
to a max resistance at 15 minutes in (step 15). Then,
repeat in reverse order for a total of 29 minutes. Try to
keep the elliptical at or above 50–60 strides per minute.
Once you are unable to maintain this, start to reduce the
resistance in reverse order each minute.

77
ROWER PYRAMID WORKOUT

1–10–1 Pyramid: Resistance Rowing

Workout on the rowing machine for 1 minute at a starting resistance level. This is step 1 of the pyramid. After each minute/step, increase the resistance by 1–2 levels, to a max resistance at 10 minutes in (step 10). Then, repeat in reverse order for a total of 20 minutes. This 20 minute rowing workout will start off easy and build up with either resistance or strokes per minute by the tenth minute. You can increase resistance or speed until the tenth minute then repeat in reverse order back to where you started.

78
SWIM SPEED INTERVAL LADDER

Warm-Up
Swim 500 meters at warm-up pace – any stroke/stretch

5–1 Ladder: Swim Intervals
The goal of this ladder is to start at 500 meters, then decrease the distance swum at each step while keeping things challenging through changing intensities. Start by swimming 5 sets of 100 meters at sprint pace. Then, swim 2 sets of 200 meters at goal pace. Next, swim 3 sets of 100 meters at sprint pace. Then, swim 1 set of 200 meters at easy pace. Finally, swim 100 meters at sprint pace for a total of 1500 meters.

79
SWIM SPEED INTERVAL LADDER: VARIATION

5–1 Ladder: Swim Intervals

The goal of this ladder is to start at 500 meters, then decrease the distance swum at each step while keeping things challenging through changing intensities. Start by swimming 1 set of 500 meters at CSS warm-up pace, timed. Then, 400 meters hypox at 8–10 strokes per breath. Next, swim 3 sets of 100 meters at CSS goal pace. Then, swim 1 set of 200 meters at CSS sprint pace. Finally, swim 100 meters (any stroke) at sprint pace for a total of 1500 meters.

Cooldown

Swim 500 meters with fins

80
MIXED SWIM LADDER

5–1 Ladder: Mixed Swim

The goal of this ladder is to start at 500 meters, then decrease the distance swum at each step while keeping things challenging through changing intensities. Start by swimming 1 set of 500 meters at warm-up pace, any stroke. Then, 400 meters freestyle at 6–8 strokes per breath. Next, swim 300 meters at CSS goal pace (shoot for 5 minutes). Then, swim 200 meters freestyle at 6–8 strokes per breath. Finally, swim 100 meters (any stroke) as fast as you can, for a total of 1500 meters.

Cooldown

Swim 500 meters with fins

81
15 LAP SWIM LADDER

Warm-Up
Swim 500 meters, timed

15 Lap Ladder: Swimming
Swim one 50-meter lap hypoxic, 6–10 strokes per breath, for each step of the ladder, starting at step 1. For each step of the ladder, increase the number of laps by 1, up to a total of 15 laps at step 15, or a total of 6000 meters.

Cooldown
Swim 5 sets of 25 meter underwaters
Rest 20 seconds

82
TRACK/FIELD TIMED PYRAMID

1–7–1 Pyramid: Timed Track

The goal of this pyramid is to run 400 meters each step of the pyramid, decreasing your lap time with each additional step. Start by running 400 meters in 2 minutes. Rest for 2 minutes, then run 400 meters again, looking to decrease your rest/running time by 10 seconds each step. Continue until you reach 400 meters in 1 minute at step 7, or until failure, then repeat in reverse order.

83
100 METER EVENTS LADDER

1–5 Ladder: 100 Meter Events
Perform 10 reps of 100 meter sprints for each step of the
ladder, starting at step 1 and progressing to step 5. Run
100 meters in between each set, for a total of 100 reps
and 400 meters run.

84
100 FLIGHTS OF STAIRS PYRAMID

1–10–1 Pyramid: Stair Climbs
For each step of the pyramid, climb 1 flight of stairs at a
run, starting with 1 flight at step 1. Progress up the
pyramid to 10 flights of stairs at step 10, then repeat in
reverse order back to 1 for a total of 100 flights of stairs.
Feel free to add "rest exercises" in between sets such
as leg stretches, abs of choice, 1 minute plank pose, etc.

85
RUNNING FOR DISTANCE
REVERSE LADDER

8–1 Reverse Ladder: Distance Running
Run 1 mile warm-up and stretch
Run ¾ mile at goal 1.5 mile pace
Run ½ mile as fast as you can
Run ¼ mile at goal mile pace
Run 300 meters timed – fast
Run 200 meters timed – faster
Run 100 meters timed – faster still
Run 50 meters timed – fastest

86
HYPOXIC SWIM PYRAMID WITH FINS

1–6–1 Ladder: Hypoxic Swimming

At each step of the pyramid, swim 100 meters freestyle at fast pace, increasing the number of strokes per breath by 2 for each new step of the pyramid. Progress up the ladder to step 6, where you'll be swimming 100 meters fast at 12 strokes per breath. Repeat in reverse order.

87
BIKE TABATA INTERVALS WITH PYRAMIDING RESISTANCE

Repeat 20 times
Each minute, increase bike resistance by 1–2 levels:
Bike 20 seconds at sprint pace
Bike 10 seconds at easy pace

88
FOOTBALL FIELD SUICIDE PYRAMID

1–10 Ladder/Pyramid: Football Field Sprints

For each step in the pyramid, sprint 10 yards out from the starting line of a football field, then sprint back. Progress up the pyramid, increasing the distance out and back by 10 yards for each step, to a max of 100 yards out and back at step 10. You can either call it here, or repeat in reverse order back down to 10 yards out/back for added challenge. For even more challenge, add an exercise every lap (push-ups, burpee, burpees, sit-ups, etc.) in either a pyramid fashion of reps or sets of 10.

89
RUN/SWIM PT LADDER

1–5 Ladder: Swim/Run PT

Step 1: Swim 100 meters OR run 400 meters, then 1 minute push-ups/plank pose

Step 2: Swim 150 meters OR Run 600 meters, then 2 minutes of push-ups/plank pose

Step 3: Swim 200 meters OR Run 800 meters, then 3 minutes of push-ups/plank pose

Step 4: Swim 250 meters OR Run 1200 meters, then 4 minutes of push-ups/plank pose

Step 5: Swim 300 meters OR run 1600 meters, then 5 minutes of push-ups/plank pose

Cooldown

Swim 500 meters OR Run 1.5 miles

Tactical Fitness Physical Test Pyramids

90
ARMY COMBAT FITNESS TEST (CFT) PYRAMID

For this workout, we set up two stations: the first station will consist of a pull-up bar, and be used for pull-ups and leg tucks. The second station will be 25 meters away, and consist of the other equipment needed (sled, deadlift bar, kettlebells or dumbbells). Each step of the pyramid will feature events at both stations, as well as specific exercises to be performed as you travel between stations.

Warm-Up
Run 1 mile, easy pace

1–10–1 Pyramid: Army CFT
Perform 1 pull-up and 1 leg tuck/knee-up for each step of the pyramid, starting at step 1. Sprint 25 meters to the deadlift bar, then perform 1 deadlift (on every odd set) and 2 hand release push-ups (on every set) for each step of the pyramid. Finally, perform one of the travel events listed below on your way back to the pull-up bar. This cycle constitutes one full step of the pyramid. Continue to progress up the pyramid until you fail or reach 10 sets, then repeat in reverse order for a total of 100 pull-ups, 100 leg tucks/knee-ups, 55 deadlifts and 200 hand release push-ups, along with 38 sets (or 950 meters) of travel exercises.

Travel Events

Choose one of the following as you travel the 25 meters to the next station:

Sprint 25 meters

100 pound sled drag – 25 meters

Farmer carry – 25 meters with two 40 pound kettlebells/ dumbbells

Medicine ball throw – 25 meters

Cooldown

Run 1 mile, easy pace

91
USMC CFT/PFT PYRAMID

For this workout, we set up two stations: the first station will consist of a pull-up bar, and be used for the PT exercises. The second station will be 25–50 meters away, and will be used for exercises like agility runs, crawls, and carries/runs. Each step of the pyramid will feature events at both stations, as well as specific exercises to be performed as you travel between stations.

Warm-Up
Run 1 mile, easy pace
Run ½ mile, fast pace

1–10–1 Pyramid: USMC CFT/PFT
Perform 1 pull-up, 2 push-ups and 3 crunches (or 3 seconds plank pose) for each step of the pyramid, starting at step 1. Sprint 25–50 meters to the second station, then perform 2 ammo can push presses for each step in the pyramid. Finally, perform one of the travel events listed below on your way back to the pull-up bar. This cycle constitutes one full step of the pyramid. Continue to progress up the pyramid until you fail or reach 10 sets, then repeat in reverse order for a total of 100 pull-ups, 200 push-ups, and 300 crunches, along with 38 sets (or 950 meters) of travel exercises.

Travel Events

Choose one of the following as you travel the 25–50 meters to the next station:

Straight Sprint

Put down cones and run an agility cone zigzag course

Ammo-can carry run OR agility zigzag to PT area

Crawl (low crawl or high crawl)

Fireman carry

Injured man drag

Cooldown

Run ½ mile, fast pace

Run 1–2 miles, steady pace

92
NAVY SEAL PST PYRAMID

The pyramid version of the Navy SEAL PST is broken into a running and swimming section, just as the test is.

1–10–1 Pyramid: Swim/PT
Perform 2 push-ups and 3 sit-ups for each step of the pyramid, then swim 100–200 meters. Continue to progress up the pyramid until you fail or reach 10 sets, then repeat in reverse order for a total of 200 push-ups, 300 sit-ups and 1900–3800 meters.

1–10–1 Pyramid: Run/Pull-Ups
Perform 1 pull-up for each step of the pyramid, then run 400 meters. Continue to progress up the pyramid until you fail or reach 10 sets, then repeat in reverse order for a total of 100 pull-ups and 7600 meters. Alternatively, you can format this as a 1–20 ladder, increasing your reps of pull-ups by 1 for each set. You can also play with the running element, doing 800 meters every other set, so long as you accumulate the needed distance by the end.

93
TACTICAL FITNESS TEST PYRAMID 1–10 REPEATS

For this workout, we set up two stations: the first station will consist of a pull-up bar, and be used for pull-ups and leg tucks. The second station will be 25 meters away, and consist of the other equipment needed (sled, kettlebells or dumbbells). Each step of the pyramid will feature events at both stations, as well as specific exercises to be performed as you travel between stations. Try this one with a 20 lbs. weight vest for more challenging calisthenics events.

1–10 Pyramid: Tactical Fitness Test Repeats

Perform 1 pull-up and 1 hanging knee-up for each step of the pyramid, starting at step 1. Sprint 25 meters to the other station and perform 2 push-ups (with 30 seconds plank hold) and 3 kettlebell swings or snatches for each step of the pyramid, starting at step 1. Finally, perform one of the travel events listed below on your way back to the pull-up bar. This cycle constitutes one full step of the pyramid. Continue to progress up the pyramid until you fail or reach 10 sets, for a total of then repeat in reverse order for a total of 55 pull-ups, 55 hanging knee-ups, 110 push-ups and 165 kettlebell movements. Repeat the entire pyramid a second time, starting from step 1, then repeat a third time if able. Stop when you fail at 1–2 events.

Travel Events

Choose one of the following as you travel the 25 meters to the next station, mixing it up each set:

[Continued on next page]

Sprint or shuttle run – 25 meters
Agility cone zig-zag course – 25 meters
Farmer walks – 25 meters carrying 1 kettlebell
Sled Pull – 25 meters

94
THE FBI FITNESS TEST PYRAMID

1–10–1 Pyramid: FBI Fitness Test

Perform 1 pull-up, 2 push-ups and 3 sit-ups for each step of the pyramid. Then, run 400 meters at your goal mile pace. Continue to progress up the pyramid until you fail or reach 10 sets, running 400 meters at goal mile pace between each set. Then, repeat the steps in reverse order; however, instead of running 400 meters between each set on the way down the pyramid, you will sprint 300 meters at fast pace every *other* set. At completion, you will have performed 100 pull-ups, 200 push-ups and 300 sit-ups, run 4000 meters and sprinted 1500 meters.

95
UPPER BODY ROUND ROBIN (UBRR) TEST PYRAMID

1–10–1 Pyramid: Pull-up/Push-up/Burpees

Perform 1 pull-up, 2 push-ups (fast pace), 2 sit-ups and 2 dips for each step of the pyramid. Continue to progress up the pyramid until you fail or reach 10 sets, then repeat in reverse order for a total of 100 pull-ups, 200 push-ups, 200 sit-ups and 200 dips. To properly prepare for the level expected in the UBRR, aim for a sit-up/second pace.

1–10 Ladder: Toes-to-Bar/Shuttle Run

Perform 1 toes-to-bar for each step of the ladder, starting from step 1. After each step, shuttle run 25 meters away and back to the pull-up bar at a fast pace. Progress from step 1 to 10, continuing to shuttle run between every step, for a total of 55 toes-to-bars and 500 meters shuttle run.

1–10 Ladder: Toes-to-Bar/Shuttle Run

Perform 2 bench presses for each step of the ladder, starting from step 1. After each step, rest with a body weight rope climb. Progress from step 1 to 10 for a total of 110 bench presses.

Run or ruck 5 miles

96
NAVY SEAL TACTICAL ATHLETE PROGRAM (TAP TEST) LADDERS

1–10/10–1 Ladder: Weighted Pull-ups/Deadlifts
Perform 1 pull-up (wearing a 25 pound weight vest) and 10 deadlifts. For each step in the ladder, *increase* the number of pull-ups by 1 and *decrease* the number of deadlifts by 1. Continue to progress up the ladder to step 10, where you will perform 10 pull-ups and 1 deadlift. On every other step, add in 2 sets of 25-yard shuttle runs, for a total of 250 yards.

1–10 Ladder: Bench Press/Long Jump
Perform 1 bench press (body weight). For each step of the ladder, you will increase your total number of reps by 1. On odd sets, perform 1 long jump, increasing the number of long jumps by 1 rep each time you perform the exercise. On even sets, perform a 5–10–5 yard shuttle run. Continue to progress to step 10, for a total of 55 bench presses, 15 long jumps and 5 shuttle runs.

Cooldown
Run 3 miles
Swim 800 meters

Pyramid
Cooldowns

97
UPPER BODY COOLDOWN REVERSE LADDER

10–1 Reverse Ladder: Upper Body Cooldown

Jog at an easy pace with dynamic stretches for 25–50 meters, then perform 1 push-up for each step of the ladder, starting with 10 push-ups at step 10. Progress down the ladder to step 1, for a total of 250–500 meters jogged and 55 push-ups. This cooldown works well after an upper body push workout or high repetition push-up/dips calisthenics.

98
LOWER BODY COOLDOWN REVERSE LADDER

10–1 Reverse Ladder: Lower Body Cooldown
Jog at an easy pace with dynamic stretches for 25–50 meters, then perform 1 burpee for each step of the ladder, starting with 10 burpees at step 10. Progress down the ladder to step 1, for a total of 250–500 meters jogged and 55 burpees. This cooldown works well after a leg day, regardless of whether the workout is a lift workout, run workout, or high repetition calisthenics workout.

99
FULL BODY COOLDOWN REVERSE LADDER

5–1 Reverse Ladder: Full Body Cooldown

Run 100 yards, then perform 1 burpee for each step of the ladder, starting with 5 burpees at step 5. Progress down the ladder to step 1, for a total of 500 yards and 15 burpees. Mix in some stretches as desired in between sets. A full body cooldown can be too much after a tough, high volume workout, so if you prefer not to do burpees for your full body exercise, you can mix in some push-ups, and even start off at a lower level of the pyramid.

100
CARDIO COOLDOWN
REVERSE LADDER

10–1 Reverse Ladder: Cardio Cooldown

Select your preferred cardio machine and work at a
reasonable intensity level for a cooldown workout. After
each minute, decrease the intensity of the workout
in whatever fashion is appropriate to the equipment
(decreasing speed, resistance, or elevation). Continue
for 5–10 minutes. The pyramid aspect of this cooldown
will help remind you to actually downshift each minute
to create a steady decreasing effort and actually cool
yourself down after a workout.

An example of this would be:
Level 10 - 1 minute
Level 8 - 1 minute
Level 6 - 1 minute
Level 4 - 1 minute
Level 2 - 1 minute
Static stretches as needed

101
SWIM WORKOUT COOLDOWN TIMED PYRAMID

After a tough swim workout, especially going 1–2 miles with fins, a good way to cooldown from the leg exertion is to mix in some aqua-jogging, treading, and dynamic stretches in the pool. Here is a 15 minute cardio cooldown that will help with breaking up any soreness.

Step 1: 5 minutes run in place in chest deep water (mix in some jumping jacks as well)

Step 2: 4 minutes dynamic stretches in chest deep water (leg swings, high knees, etc.)

Step 3: 3 minutes tread water (mix in a combination of arms only and legs only)

Step 4: 2 minutes tread water (legs only, multiple kicks)

Step 5: 1 minute mix bottom bounce using arms only (similar to jumping jacks) to go up/down in deep end

RESOURCES

HEROES OF TOMORROW

We do local training for FREE in the Annapolis/Severna Park, MD area year-round. Our weekly schedule can be found at the Heroes of Tomorrow page. Check in with us prior to attending and fill out the questionnaire on the page above.

ONLINE COACHING

If you need personal training help, check out the StewSmithFitness.com website where you can train with me through our Online Coaching program.

FAQS

Contact us at stew@stewsmith.com if you have any questions about training, specific workouts, or if you would like more information on how to attend our local workouts, make bulk purchases, or find online coaching resources.

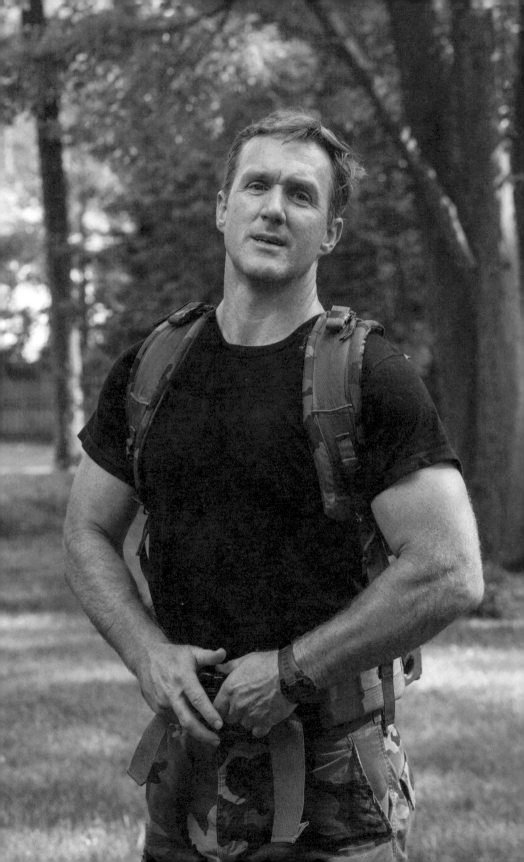

ABOUT THE AUTHOR

Stew Smith, CSCS, is a professional fitness writer with over 20 years of experience in the special ops, military, law enforcement, and firefighting fitness genre, also known as "tactical fitness."

Stew Smith develops fitness training routines that mimic job-related events a tactical operator will need to be successful in training and when operational. Drawing from his Navy SEAL experiences and life-long education and experiences in athletics, preparation for training, as well as coaching others, Stew Smith has developed programs that not only physically prepare you for the tactical life, but also prepare you to deal with everyday issues that require strength, speed, agility, muscle stamina, cardiovascular endurance, and mobility.

He is certified by the National Strength and Conditioning Association as a strength and conditioning specialist (CSCS). His books and downloadable manuals can take you from beginner to a special ops level conditioned tactical athlete. Let these workouts assist you in becoming a better conditioned athlete.

Stew Smith resides near Annapolis, Maryland, where he is actively involved with training tactical athletes who seek special operations, military, police, SWAT, and firefighting professions.

ALSO FROM STEWART SMITH